STAGE 4

KIDNEY DISEASE COOKBOOK

FOR SENIORS

28-day meal plan nutritional guide with Low Potassium, Low Phosphorus, and Low Sodium Recipes to improve your renal health

Dr. JANE THORNTHWAITE

2

TABLE OF CONTENTS

Chapter One

INTRODUCTION

Understanding Stage 4 Kidney Disease

What is Stage 4 Kidney Disease?

Stage 4 Kidney Disease is an advanced stage of chronic kidney disease characterized by a significant reduction in kidney function, leading to various symptoms and complications. It is marked by a moderate decrease in the glomerular filtration rate (GFR), with the kidneys experiencing substantial damage. Individuals at this stage may require careful management and medical intervention to address complications and slow the progression of the disease.

Dietary Challenges for Seniors with Kidney Disease

Seniors with kidney disease often face dietary challenges due to the need for specific nutritional modifications. These challenges are influenced by the necessity to manage factors such as protein intake, phosphorus and potassium levels, and fluid restriction. Addressing these dietary considerations is crucial to supporting kidney health and overall well-being in older individuals with kidney disease.

Importance of Nutrition in Managing Kidney Health

Nutrition plays a crucial role in managing kidney health, particularly for individuals with kidney disease. The importance of nutrition in this context includes:

1. **Disease Progression Control:** Proper nutrition can help slow the progression of

kidney disease by managing factors such as blood pressure, protein intake, and levels of phosphorus and potassium. Adhering to a kidney-friendly diet can alleviate stress on the kidneys and minimize further damage.

2. **Blood Pressure Regulation:** A well-balanced diet that is low in sodium can help regulate blood pressure. High blood pressure is a common complication of kidney disease, and managing it is essential to prevent additional harm to the kidneys.

3. **Protein Management:** Controlling protein intake is critical in managing kidney health. Consuming an appropriate amount of high-quality protein can help reduce the workload on the kidneys, preventing the accumulation of waste products and preserving kidney function.

4.   **Fluid Balance:** For individuals with kidney disease, maintaining an optimal fluid balance is important. Monitoring and restricting fluid intake can help prevent complications such as fluid retention and swelling.

5.   **Electrolyte Balance:** Kidneys are responsible for maintaining proper levels of electrolytes such as potassium and phosphorus. Nutrition interventions, including limiting certain foods, help prevent imbalances that can lead to complications like heart and bone issues.

6.   **Minimization of Symptomatic Effects:** Kidney disease can cause symptoms such as fatigue, anemia, and bone disorders. A well-managed diet can help minimize these symptoms, enhancing the overall quality of life for individuals with kidney disease.

7. **Customized Nutrition Plans:** Every individual's nutritional needs may vary based on the stage and specific conditions of kidney disease. Tailoring nutrition plans to individual requirements ensures that dietary recommendations address the unique challenges and goals of each person.

8. **Prevention of Nutrient Deficiencies:** Dietary restrictions associated with kidney disease may increase the risk of nutrient deficiencies. A carefully planned diet, often developed in consultation with a registered dietitian, helps prevent deficiencies and supports overall well-being.

9. **Improved Immune Function:** Proper nutrition supports a robust immune system, which is important for individuals with

kidney disease who may be more susceptible to infections.

Chapter 1

Kidney-Friendly Basics

Low-Potassium Foods:

Explanation: Potassium is a mineral that the kidneys typically help regulate. In kidney disease, impaired kidney function can lead to potassium buildup, which may result in complications like irregular heartbeats. Choosing low-potassium foods is crucial to manage potassium levels.

Examples: Apples, berries, cabbage, cauliflower, cucumber, green beans, rice, and limited portions of certain fruits.

Low-Phosphorus Alternatives:

Explanation: Phosphorus is another mineral that kidneys usually regulate. In kidney disease, phosphorus levels can become elevated, leading to bone and cardiovascular issues. Identifying and consuming low-phosphorus alternatives helps control phosphorus intake.

Examples: White bread, white rice, apples, cabbage, green beans, and egg whites. Limiting high-phosphorus foods like dairy, nuts, and certain meats is also essential.

Smart Sodium Swaps:

Explanation: High sodium intake can contribute to high blood pressure and fluid retention, both of which can worsen kidney disease. Smart sodium swaps involve choosing low-sodium alternatives and avoiding processed and salty foods.

Examples: Using herbs and spices for flavor instead of salt, choosing fresh fruits and vegetables, opting for low-sodium or no-salt-added versions of canned goods, and limiting the use of condiments high in sodium.

Balancing Proteins, Carbs, and Fats:

Explanation: Achieving a balance between proteins, carbohydrates, and fats is crucial for overall health and kidney function. For those with kidney disease, managing protein intake is particularly important to reduce the burden on the kidneys.

Examples: Opting for lean proteins like chicken and fish, incorporating plant-based protein sources, choosing whole grains for carbohydrates, and including healthy fats from sources like avocados and olive oil in moderation.

Monitoring Fluid Intake:

Explanation: Impaired kidney function can lead to difficulty in regulating fluid balance. Monitoring fluid intake is essential to prevent fluid overload and associated complications such as edema and high blood pressure.

Examples: Limiting the intake of high-fluid foods like soups, ice cream, and water-rich fruits. Tracking fluid intake and adhering to prescribed limits based on individual needs.

Chapter 2:

28-Day Sample Meal Plans for Seniors

it's important for seniors with specific health conditions, including kidney disease, to consult with a healthcare professional or a registered dietitian for personalized recommendations.

Week 1

Day 1:

Breakfast:

- Scrambled eggs with spinach
- Whole grain toast
- Orange slices

Lunch:

- Grilled chicken breast
- Quinoa salad with cucumber and cherry tomatoes
- Steamed broccoli

Dinner:

- Baked salmon
- Sweet potato wedges
- Mixed green salad

Snack:

- Greek yogurt with a handful of almonds

Beverage:

- Herbal tea or infused water

Day 2:

Breakfast:

- Oatmeal with sliced strawberries
- Boiled egg
- Whole grain toast

Lunch:

- Turkey and vegetable stir-fry
- Brown rice

Dinner:

- Lentil soup

- Baked cod fillet
- Steamed asparagus

Snack:

- Cottage cheese with pineapple chunks

Beverage:

- Decaffeinated green tea

Day 3:

Breakfast:

- Whole grain waffles with blueberries
- Greek yogurt
- Banana slices

Lunch:

- Spinach and feta stuffed chicken breast
- Quinoa and black bean salad

Dinner:

- Shrimp and vegetable kebabs
- Cauliflower rice

- Mixed greens with vinaigrette

Snack:

- Sliced apple with peanut butter

Beverage:

- Water with lemon

Day 4:

Breakfast:

- Smoothie with kale, banana, and almond milk
- Whole grain muffin

Lunch:

- Tuna salad with mixed greens
- Whole grain crackers

Dinner:

- Beef and vegetable stir-fry
- Brown rice

Snack:

- Carrot and cucumber sticks with hummus

Beverage:

- Infused water with mint and cucumber

Day 5:

Breakfast:

- Yogurt parfait with granola and berries
- Boiled egg

Lunch:

- Chicken and vegetable soup
- Quinoa and chickpea salad

Dinner:

- Baked tilapia with lemon
- Roasted sweet potatoes
- Green beans

Snack:

- Trail mix with nuts and dried fruits

Beverage:

- Herbal tea

Day 6:

Breakfast:

- Pancakes with sliced peaches
- Cottage cheese
- Herbal tea

Lunch:

- Grilled vegetable and feta wrap
- Quinoa salad

Dinner:

- Baked chicken thighs
- Brown rice
- Steamed broccoli and carrots

Snack:

- Orange slices

Beverage:

- Water with a splash of lemon

Day 7:

Breakfast:

- Scrambled tofu with tomatoes and spinach
- Whole grain toast
- Banana slices

Lunch:

- Lentil and vegetable curry
- Basmati rice

Dinner:

- Grilled salmon
- Quinoa pilaf
- Mixed green salad

Snack:

- Greek yogurt with honey

Beverage:

- Decaffeinated herbal tea

Week 2

Day 8:

Breakfast:

- Whole grain bagel with cream cheese
- Sliced melon
- Herbal tea

Lunch:

- Turkey and avocado wrap
- Quinoa salad with cherry tomatoes

Dinner:

- Baked cod with lemon and herbs
- Sweet potato mash
- Steamed green beans

Snack:

- Mixed nuts

Beverage:

- Infused water with cucumber and mint

Day 9:

Breakfast:

- Greek yogurt parfait with granola and mixed berries
- Boiled egg

Lunch:

- Chickpea and vegetable stir-fry
- Brown rice

Dinner:

- Grilled shrimp skewers
- Quinoa pilaf with peas
- Mixed green salad

Snack:

- Apple slices with almond butter

Beverage:

- Decaffeinated green tea

Day 10:

Breakfast:

- Smoothie with kale, banana, and almond milk
- Whole grain muffin

Lunch:

- Caprese salad with balsamic glaze
- Whole grain crackers

Dinner:

- Beef and broccoli stir-fry
- Basmati rice

Snack:

- Carrot and cucumber sticks with hummus

Beverage:

- Water with a splash of lemon

Day 11:

Breakfast:

- Pancakes with mixed berries

- Cottage cheese
- Herbal tea

Lunch:
- Quinoa and black bean bowl
- Avocado slices

Dinner:
- Baked chicken breasts with rosemary
- Roasted sweet potatoes
- Steamed broccoli

Snack:
- Orange slices

Beverage:
- Decaffeinated herbal tea

Day 12:

Breakfast:
- Scrambled eggs with sautéed mushrooms and spinach
- Whole grain toast
- Banana slices

Lunch:

- Lentil soup
- Whole grain roll

Dinner:

- Grilled salmon
- Quinoa salad with cucumber and cherry tomatoes
- Mixed greens with vinaigrette

Snack:

- Trail mix with nuts and dried fruits

Beverage:

- Water with a splash of lemon

Day 13:

Breakfast:

- Oatmeal with sliced strawberries
- Boiled egg

Lunch:

- Tuna salad with mixed greens
- Quinoa and chickpea salad

Dinner:

- Shrimp and vegetable kebabs
- Brown rice

Snack:

- Greek yogurt with honey

Beverage:

- Infused water with cucumber and mint

Day 14:

Breakfast:

- Whole grain waffles with blueberries
- Greek yogurt
- Herbal tea

Lunch:

- Spinach and feta stuffed chicken breast
- Quinoa salad

Dinner:

- Beef and vegetable stir-fry

- Cauliflower rice
- Mixed green salad

Snack:

- Cottage cheese with pineapple chunks

Beverage:

- Water with a splash of lemon

Week 3

Day 15:

Breakfast:

- Scrambled tofu with tomatoes and spinach
- Whole grain toast
- Orange slices

Lunch:

- Lentil and vegetable curry
- Basmati rice

Dinner:

- Grilled salmon
- Quinoa pilaf
- Mixed green salad

Snack:

- Greek yogurt with a handful of almonds

Beverage:

- Decaffeinated herbal tea

Day 16:

Breakfast:

- Whole grain bagel with cream cheese
- Sliced melon
- Herbal tea

Lunch:

- Turkey and avocado wrap
- Quinoa salad with cherry tomatoes

Dinner:

- Baked cod with lemon and herbs
- Sweet potato mash
- Steamed green beans

Snack:

- Mixed nuts

Beverage:

- Infused water with cucumber and mint

Day 17:

Breakfast:

- Greek yogurt parfait with granola and mixed berries
- Boiled egg

Lunch:

- Chickpea and vegetable stir-fry
- Brown rice

Dinner:

- Grilled shrimp skewers
- Quinoa pilaf with peas

- Mixed green salad

Snack:

- Apple slices with almond butter

Beverage:

- Water with a splash of lemon

Day 18:

Breakfast:

- Smoothie with kale, banana, and almond milk
- Whole grain muffin

Lunch:

- Caprese salad with balsamic glaze
- Whole grain crackers

Dinner:

- Beef and broccoli stir-fry
- Basmati rice

Snack:

- Carrot and cucumber sticks with hummus

Beverage:

- Decaffeinated green tea

Day 19:

Breakfast:

- Pancakes with mixed berries
- Cottage cheese
- Herbal tea

Lunch:

- Quinoa and black bean bowl
- Avocado slices

Dinner:

- Baked chicken breasts with rosemary
- Roasted sweet potatoes
- Steamed broccoli

Snack:

- Orange slices

Beverage:

- Decaffeinated herbal tea

Day 20:

Breakfast:

- Scrambled eggs with sautéed mushrooms and spinach
- Whole grain toast
- Banana slices

Lunch:

- Lentil soup
- Whole grain roll

Dinner:

- Grilled salmon
- Quinoa salad with cucumber and cherry tomatoes
- Mixed greens with vinaigrette

Snack:

- Trail mix with nuts and dried fruits

Beverage:

- Water with a splash of lemon

Day 21:

Breakfast:

- Oatmeal with sliced strawberries
- Boiled egg

Lunch:

- Tuna salad with mixed greens
- Quinoa and chickpea salad

Dinner:

- Shrimp and vegetable kebabs
- Brown rice

Snack:

- Greek yogurt with honey

Beverage:

- Infused water with cucumber and mint

Week 4

Day 22:

Breakfast:

- Whole grain waffles with blueberries
- Greek yogurt
- Herbal tea

Lunch:

- Spinach and feta stuffed chicken breast
- Quinoa salad

Dinner:

- Beef and vegetable stir-fry
- Cauliflower rice
- Mixed green salad

Snack:

- Cottage cheese with pineapple chunks

Beverage:

- Water with a splash of lemon

Day 23:

Breakfast:

- Scrambled tofu with tomatoes and spinach
- Whole grain toast
- Orange slices

Lunch:

- Lentil and vegetable curry
- Basmati rice

Dinner:

- Grilled salmon
- Quinoa pilaf
- Mixed green salad

Snack:

- Greek yogurt with a handful of almonds

Beverage:

- Decaffeinated herbal tea

Day 24:

Breakfast:

- Whole grain bagel with cream cheese
- Sliced melon
- Herbal tea

Lunch:

- Turkey and avocado wrap
- Quinoa salad with cherry tomatoes

Dinner:

- Baked cod with lemon and herbs
- Sweet potato mash
- Steamed green beans

Snack:

- Mixed nuts

Beverage:

- Infused water with cucumber and mint

Day 25:

Breakfast:

- Greek yogurt parfait with granola and mixed berries
- Boiled egg

Lunch:

- Chickpea and vegetable stir-fry
- Brown rice

Dinner:

- Grilled shrimp skewers
- Quinoa pilaf with peas
- Mixed green salad

Snack:

- Apple slices with almond butter

Beverage:

- Water with a splash of lemon

Day 26:

Breakfast:

- Smoothie with kale, banana, and almond milk
- Whole grain muffin

Lunch:

- Caprese salad with balsamic glaze
- Whole grain crackers

Dinner:

- Beef and broccoli stir-fry
- Basmati rice

Snack:

- Carrot and cucumber sticks with hummus

Beverage:

- Decaffeinated green tea

Day 27:

Breakfast:

- Pancakes with mixed berries

- Cottage cheese
- Herbal tea

Lunch:

- Quinoa and black bean bowl
- Avocado slices

Dinner:

- Baked chicken breasts with rosemary
- Roasted sweet potatoes
- Steamed broccoli

Snack:

- Orange slices

Beverage:

- Decaffeinated herbal tea

Day 28:

Breakfast:

- Scrambled eggs with sautéed mushrooms and spinach
- Whole grain toast
- Banana slices

Lunch:

- Lentil soup
- Whole grain roll

Dinner:

- Grilled salmon
- Quinoa salad with cucumber and cherry tomatoes
- Mixed greens with vinaigrette

Snack:

- Trail mix with nuts and dried fruits

Beverage:

- Water with a splash of lemon

Dining Out Strategies

Here are some strategies for seniors with kidney disease when dining out:

1. **Review the Menu in Advance:**

Many restaurants now provide their menus online. Reviewing the menu beforehand allows individuals to identify kidney-friendly options and plan their choices.

2. **Choose Grilled or Baked Proteins:**

Opt for grilled or baked protein options, such as fish or chicken, rather than fried or heavily seasoned choices. Request minimal added salt during preparation.

3. **Ask for Modifications:**

Don't hesitate to ask the waiter for modifications to your dish. For example, request sauces or dressings on the side to control sodium intake.

4. **Be Mindful of Portion Sizes:**

Restaurant portions are often larger than necessary. Consider sharing a dish with a dining companion or ask for a takeout container at the beginning of the meal to save half for later.

5. **Choose Low-Phosphorus Sides:**

Opt for sides that are low in phosphorus. This might include steamed vegetables, plain rice, or a baked potato without excessive toppings.

6. **Limit High-Potassium Foods:**

Be cautious of high-potassium ingredients like tomatoes, avocados, and potatoes. Choose dishes with kidney-friendly alternatives or ask for substitutions.

7. **Request Nutritional Information:**

Some restaurants provide nutritional information for their dishes upon request. Knowing the nutritional content helps in making informed choices about potassium, phosphorus, and sodium content.

8. **Beware of Hidden Sodium:**

Restaurant meals often contain hidden sodium. Be cautious of condiments, sauces, and dressings, as they can significantly contribute to sodium intake.

9. **Choose Kidney-Friendly Beverages:**
Opt for water, herbal tea, or other low-sugar, low-sodium beverages instead of sugary drinks or those high in caffeine.

10. **Communicate Dietary Restrictions:**
Inform the waiter about any dietary restrictions or preferences, especially if you have specific health conditions like kidney disease. Most restaurants are willing to accommodate dietary needs.

11. **Consider Ethnic Cuisine:**
Some ethnic cuisines offer kidney-friendly options. For example, Japanese or Mediterranean restaurants may have dishes that align with dietary recommendations for kidney health.

12. Practice Portion Control:

If the restaurant serves large portions, consider ordering an appetizer or a small entrée. This allows for better control over portion sizes.

13. Bring Medications If Needed:

If you take medications related to your kidney condition, ensure you have them with you. If dining out during medication times, plan accordingly.

Chapter 3

Breakfast Delights

Oatmeal with Berries and Almonds:

Ingredients:

- Rolled oats
- Mixed berries (blueberries, strawberries)
- Chopped almonds

Instructions:

1. Cook oats according to package instructions. Top with mixed berries and chopped almonds.

Nutritional Information (per serving):

1. Calories: 250
2. Protein: 8g
3. Potassium: 150mg
4. Phosphorus: 100mg

Vegetable Omelette:

Ingredients:

1. Eggs
2. Spinach
3. Bell peppers
4. Onion

Instructions:

1. Whisk eggs and pour into a hot, non-stick pan. Add chopped vegetables, and cook until set.

Nutritional Information (per serving):

- Calories: 200
- Protein: 15g
- Potassium: 200mg
- Phosphorus: 150mg

Greek Yogurt Parfait:

Ingredients:

1. Greek yogurt
2. Granola

3. Sliced strawberries

Instructions:

1. Layer Greek yogurt with granola and sliced strawberries.

Nutritional Information (per serving):

1. Calories: 180

2. Protein: 15g

3. Potassium: 180mg

4. Phosphorus: 120mg

Smoothie Bowl:

Ingredients:

1. Frozen mixed berries

2. Banana

3. Spinach

4. Almond milk

Instructions:

1. Blend berries, bananas, and spinach with almond milk. Top with sliced almonds.

Nutritional Information (per serving):

1. Calories: 220
2. Protein: 8g
3. Potassium: 250mg
4. Phosphorus: 100mg

Low-Phosphorus Pancakes:

Ingredients:

1. Whole wheat flour
2. Almond milk
3. Egg substitute

Instructions:

1. Mix ingredients, and cook pancakes on a non-stick griddle. Serve with a small amount of syrup.

Nutritional Information (per serving):

1. Calories: 180
2. Protein: 6g
3. Potassium: 120mg
4. Phosphorus: 70mg

Egg White Scramble with Spinach and Tomatoes:

Ingredients:

1. Egg whites
2. Fresh spinach
3. Cherry tomatoes

Instructions:

1. Cook egg whites, then add chopped spinach and tomatoes.

Nutritional Information (per serving):

1. Calories: 120
2. Protein: 15g
3. Potassium: 180mg
4. Phosphorus: 100mg

Quinoa Breakfast Bowl:

Ingredients:

1. Quinoa
2. Sliced peaches
3. Slivered almonds

Instructions:

1. Cook quinoa and top with sliced peaches and slivered almonds.

Nutritional Information (per serving):

1. Calories: 220
2. Protein: 8g
3. Potassium: 200mg
4. Phosphorus: 150mg

Apple Cinnamon Baked Oatmeal:

Ingredients:

1. Rolled oats
2. Apples
3. Cinnamon

Instructions:

1. Mix oats, diced apples, and cinnamon. Bake until golden brown.

Nutritional Information (per serving):

1. Calories: 240
2. Protein: 6g

3. Potassium: 180mg

4. Phosphorus: 100mg

Chia Seed Pudding:

Ingredients:

1. Chia seeds

2. Unsweetened almond milk

3. Fresh berries

Instructions:

Mix chia seeds with almond milk and refrigerate. Top with fresh berries before serving.

Nutritional Information (per serving):

1. Calories: 180

2. Protein: 5g

3. Potassium: 120mg

4. Phosphorus: 80mg

Whole Grain Toast with Avocado and Radish Slices:

Ingredients:

1. Whole grain bread
2. Avocado
3. Radishes

Instructions:

1. Toast the bread, spread with mashed avocado, and top with radish slices.

Nutritional Information (per serving):

1. Calories: 160
2. Protein: 4g
3. Potassium: 250mg
4. Phosphorus: 90mg

Mango and Banana Smoothie:

Ingredients:

1. Frozen mango
2. Banana
3. Almond milk

Instructions:

1. Blend frozen mango, banana, and almond milk until smooth.

Nutritional Information (per serving):

- Calories: 150
- Protein: 3g
- Potassium: 240mg
- Phosphorus: 70mg

Whole Grain English Muffin with Smoked Salmon:

Ingredients:

1. Whole grain English muffin
2. Smoked salmon
3. Cream cheese (low-sodium)

Instructions:

Toast the English muffin, spread with low-sodium cream cheese and top with smoked salmon.

Nutritional Information (per serving):

1. Calories: 220
2. Protein: 15g
3. Potassium: 180mg
4. Phosphorus: 150mg

Pear and Walnut Breakfast Salad:

Ingredients:

1. Mixed greens
2. Sliced pears
3. Chopped walnuts

Instructions:

Toss mixed greens with sliced pears and chopped walnuts. Drizzle with balsamic vinaigrette.

Nutritional Information (per serving):

1. Calories: 190
2. Protein: 4g
3. Potassium: 220mg
4. Phosphorus: 80mg

Blueberry Muffins (Low-Phosphorus):

Ingredients:

1. Whole wheat flour
2. Fresh or frozen blueberries
3. Almond milk

Instructions:

Mix ingredients, pour into muffin cups, and bake until a toothpick comes out clean.

Nutritional Information (per serving):

1. Calories: 180
2. Protein: 5g
3. Potassium: 120mg
4. Phosphorus: 70mg

Chapter 4

Lunch for Kidney Health

Grilled Lemon Herb Chicken:

Ingredients:

- Chicken breast
- Lemon juice
- Fresh herbs (rosemary, thyme)

Instructions:

Marinate chicken in lemon juice and herbs.

Grill until cooked through.

Nutritional Information (per serving):

- Calories: 220
- Protein: 25g
- Potassium: 270mg
- Phosphorus: 150mg

Quinoa and Black Bean Salad:

Ingredients:

- Quinoa

- Black beans
- Cherry tomatoes

Instructions:

Cook quinoa, and mix with black beans and cherry tomatoes.

Nutritional Information (per serving):

- Calories: 200
- Protein: 8g
- Potassium: 180mg
- Phosphorus: 120mg

Salmon and Vegetable Stir-Fry:

Ingredients:

- Salmon fillet
- Broccoli
- Bell peppers

Instructions:

- Stir-fry salmon and vegetables in low-sodium sauce.

Nutritional Information (per serving):

- Calories: 250
- Protein: 20g
- Potassium: 300mg
- Phosphorus: 200mg

Turkey and Avocado Wrap:

Ingredients:

- Whole grain wrap
- Turkey slices
- Avocado

Instructions:

Assemble the wrap with turkey and sliced avocado.

Nutritional Information (per serving):

- Calories: 280
- Protein: 20g
- Potassium: 250mg
- Phosphorus: 150mg

Eggplant and Tomato Pasta:

Ingredients:

- Whole wheat pasta
- Eggplant
- Tomatoes

Instructions:

Roast eggplant and tomatoes, and toss with cooked pasta.

Nutritional Information (per serving):

- Calories: 230
- Protein: 8g
- Potassium: 200mg
- Phosphorus: 120mg

Chicken and Vegetable Quinoa Bowl:

Ingredients:

- Cooked quinoa
- Grilled chicken
- Mixed vegetables (zucchini, carrots)

Instructions:

Combine quinoa, grilled chicken, and mixed vegetables.

Nutritional Information (per serving):

- Calories: 260
- Protein: 22g
- Potassium: 230mg
- Phosphorus: 150mg

Lentil and Vegetable Curry:

Ingredients:

- Lentils
- Mixed Vegetables
- Curry spices

Instructions:

- Cook lentils with mixed vegetables and curry spices.

Nutritional Information (per serving):

- Calories: 220
- Protein: 15g

- Potassium: 270mg
- Phosphorus: 180mg

Spinach and Feta Stuffed Chicken Breast:

Ingredients:

- Chicken breast
- Fresh spinach
- Feta cheese

Instructions:

Stuff chicken breast with spinach and feta, and bake until cooked.

Nutritional Information (per serving):

- Calories: 240
- Protein: 25g
- Potassium: 260mg
- Phosphorus: 150mg

Cauliflower Fried Rice:

Ingredients:

- Cauliflower rice

- Peas
- Carrots

Instructions:

Stir-fry cauliflower rice with peas and carrots.

Nutritional Information (per serving):

- Calories: 180
- Protein: 7g
- Potassium: 200mg
- Phosphorus: 120mg

Tuna Salad with Mixed Greens:

Ingredients:

- Canned tuna (in water)
- Mixed greens
- Cherry tomatoes

Instructions:

Combine tuna with mixed greens and cherry tomatoes.

Nutritional Information (per serving):

- Calories: 200
- Protein: 20g
- Potassium: 250mg
- Phosphorus: 150mg

Grilled Shrimp and Quinoa Pilaf:

Ingredients:

- Shrimp
- Quinoa
- Vegetables (bell peppers, onions)
  1. *Instructions:*

Grill shrimp and serve over quinoa pilaf with sautéed vegetables.

Nutritional Information (per serving):

- Calories: 250
- Protein: 18g
- Potassium: 280mg
- Phosphorus: 200mg

Mushroom and Brown Rice Risotto:

Ingredients:

- Brown rice
- Mushrooms
- Low-sodium vegetable broth

Instructions:

Cook brown rice with mushrooms and vegetable broth.

- *Nutritional Information (per serving):*
  - Calories: 210
  - Protein: 7g
  - Potassium: 180mg
  - Phosphorus: 120mg

Baked Cod with Lemon and Herbs:

Ingredients:

- Cod fillet
- Lemon juice
- Fresh herbs (parsley, dill)

Instructions:

Marinate cod with lemon and herbs, and bake until flaky.

Nutritional Information (per serving):

- Calories: 220
- Protein: 25g
- Potassium: 250mg
- Phosphorus: 180mg

Turkey and Vegetable Stir-Fry:

Ingredients:

- Ground turkey
- Stir-fry vegetables (broccoli, snap peas)
- Low-sodium soy sauce

Instructions:

- Cook ground turkey with stir-fry vegetables and soy sauce.
- *Nutritional Information (per serving):*

- Calories: 230
- Protein: 20g
- Potassium: 280mg
- Phosphorus: 150mg

Roasted Sweet Potatoes and Chickpea Salad:

Ingredients:

- Sweet potatoes
- Chickpeas
- Olive oil, herbs

Instructions:

Roast sweet potatoes and chickpeas, and toss with olive oil and herbs.

Nutritional Information (per serving):

- Calories: 210
- Protein: 6g
- Potassium: 300mg
- Phosphorus: 150mg

Chapter 5

Dinner Delicacies

Baked Chicken Thighs with Rosemary:

Ingredients:

- Chicken thighs
- Fresh rosemary
- Garlic

Instructions:

Rub chicken thighs with chopped rosemary and minced garlic. Bake until golden.

Nutritional Information (per serving):

- Calories: 250
- Protein: 28g
- Potassium: 300mg
- Phosphorus: 180mg

Grilled Salmon with Lemon and Dill:

Ingredients:

- Salmon fillet
- Lemon juice
- Fresh dill

Instructions:

Marinate salmon with lemon juice and dill. Grill until flaky.

Nutritional Information (per serving):

- Calories: 280
- Protein: 25g
- Potassium: 320mg
- Phosphorus: 200mg

Mushroom and Spinach Stuffed Bell Peppers:

Ingredients:

- Bell peppers
- Mushrooms
- Spinach

Instructions:

Sauté mushrooms and spinach, and stuff into bell peppers. Bake until tender.

Nutritional Information (per serving):

- Calories: 220
- Protein: 12g
- Potassium: 250mg
- Phosphorus: 150mg

Lemon Garlic Shrimp Skewers:

Ingredients:

- Shrimp
- Lemon zest
- Garlic

Instructions:

Thread shrimp onto skewers, and season with lemon zest and minced garlic. Grill until cooked.

Nutritional Information (per serving):

- Calories: 230

- Protein: 20g
- Potassium: 280mg
- Phosphorus: 180mg

Vegetarian Chili:

Ingredients:

- Kidney beans
- Black beans
- Tomatoes

Instructions:

Cook kidney beans, black beans, and tomatoes with chili spices.

Nutritional Information (per serving):

- Calories: 240
- Protein: 15g
- Potassium: 300mg
- Phosphorus: 180mg

Baked Cod with Tomato and Basil:

Ingredients:

- Cod fillet
- Tomatoes
- Fresh basil

Instructions:

Top cod with sliced tomatoes and chopped basil. Bake until the fish is flaky.

Nutritional Information (per serving):

- Calories: 250
- Protein: 25g
- Potassium: 280mg
- Phosphorus: 200mg

Quinoa and Vegetable Stir-Fry:

Ingredients:

- Quinoa
- Mixed vegetables (broccoli, bell peppers)
- Low-sodium soy sauce

Instructions:

Cook quinoa, stir-fry vegetables, and toss with low-sodium soy sauce.

Nutritional Information (per serving):

- Calories: 230
- Protein: 10g
- Potassium: 250mg
- Phosphorus: 150mg

Roasted Chicken Drumsticks with Herbs:

Ingredients:

- Chicken drumsticks
- Mixed herbs (thyme, oregano)
- Olive oil

Instructions:

Coat drumsticks with herbs and olive oil. Roast until crispy.

Nutritional Information (per serving):

- Calories: 260
- Protein: 30g

- Potassium: 320mg
- Phosphorus: 180mg

Eggplant Parmesan:

Ingredients:

- Eggplant
- Low-sodium marinara sauce
- Mozzarella cheese

Instructions:

Layer sliced eggplant with marinara sauce and mozzarella. Bake until bubbly.

Nutritional Information (per serving):

- Calories: 240
- Protein: 10g
- Potassium: 270mg
- Phosphorus: 150mg

Turkey and Vegetable Skewers:

Ingredients:

- Ground turkey

- Zucchini
- Cherry tomatoes

Instructions:

Form ground turkey into skewers with zucchini and tomatoes. Grill until cooked.

Nutritional Information (per serving):

- Calories: 230
- Protein: 20g
- Potassium: 250mg
- Phosphorus: 180mg

Cauliflower and Chickpea Curry:

Ingredients:

- Cauliflower
- Chickpeas
- Curry spices

Instructions:

Cook cauliflower and chickpeas with curry spices.

Nutritional Information (per serving):

- Calories: 220
- Protein: 10g
- Potassium: 270mg
- Phosphorus: 150mg

Salmon and Asparagus Foil Packets:

Ingredients:

- Salmon fillet
- Asparagus
- Lemon slices

Instructions:

Place salmon, asparagus, and lemon slices in foil packets. Bake until the salmon is cooked.

Nutritional Information (per serving):

- Calories: 270
- Protein: 25g
- Potassium: 320mg
- Phosphorus: 200mg

Lentil Soup:

Ingredients:

- Lentils
- Carrots
- Celery

Instructions:

Cook lentils with carrots and celery in a low-sodium broth.

Nutritional Information (per serving):

- Calories: 210
- Protein: 15g
- Potassium: 250mg
- Phosphorus: 180mg

Vegetable and Chicken Sauté:

Ingredients:

- Chicken breast
- Mixed vegetables (bell peppers, snap peas)
- Olive oil

Instructions:

Sauté chicken and vegetables in olive oil until cooked.

Nutritional Information (per serving):

- Calories: 240

- Protein: 25g

- Potassium: 280mg

- Phosphorus: 150mg

Shrimp and Vegetable Skillet:

Ingredients:

- Shrimp

- Mixed vegetables (zucchini, cherry tomatoes)

- Garlic

Instructions:

Sauté shrimp and vegetables with minced garlic until shrimp is pink.

Nutritional Information (per serving):

- Calories: 230
- Protein: 20g
- Potassium: 270mg
- Phosphorus: 180mg

Chapter 6

Snacks and Desserts

Snacks:

Cucumber and Hummus Bites:

Ingredients:

- Cucumber slices
- Hummus

Instructions:

Top cucumber slices with a dollop of hummus.

Nutritional Information (per serving):

- Calories: 50
- Protein: 2g
- Potassium: 120mg
- Phosphorus: 40mg

Greek Yogurt with Berries:

Ingredients:

- Greek yogurt
- Mixed berries

Instructions:

Mix Greek yogurt with fresh berries.

Nutritional Information (per serving):

- Calories: 120
- Protein: 10g
- Potassium: 150mg
- Phosphorus: 80mg

Rice Cake with Almond Butter:

Ingredients:

- Brown rice cake
- Almond butter (unsalted)

Instructions:

Spread almond butter on a rice cake.

Nutritional Information (per serving):

- Calories: 100
- Protein: 3g
- Potassium: 80mg
- Phosphorus: 60mg

Deviled Eggs:

Ingredients:

- Hard-boiled eggs
- Greek yogurt
- Mustard

Instructions:

Mix egg yolks with Greek yogurt and mustard. Fill egg whites.

Nutritional Information (per serving):

- Calories: 70
- Protein: 6g
- Potassium: 70mg
- Phosphorus: 80mg

Cottage Cheese with Pineapple:

Ingredients:

- Low-fat cottage cheese
- Pineapple chunks

Instructions:

Combine cottage cheese with pineapple chunks.

Nutritional Information (per serving):

- Calories: 120
- Protein: 15g
- Potassium: 150mg
- Phosphorus: 100mg

Vegetable Sticks with Tzatziki:

Ingredients:

- Carrot and cucumber sticks
- Tzatziki sauce (low-sodium)

Instructions:

Dip vegetable sticks into tzatziki sauce.

Nutritional Information (per serving):

- Calories: 50
- Protein: 2g
- Potassium: 70mg
- Phosphorus: 40mg

Mixed Nuts:

Ingredients:

Almonds, walnuts, and pistachios (unsalted)

Instructions:

Mix a variety of unsalted nuts for a crunchy snack.

Nutritional Information (per serving):

- Calories: 180
- Protein: 6g
- Potassium: 200mg
- Phosphorus: 120mg

Desserts:

Baked Apples with Cinnamon:

Ingredients:

- Apples
- Cinnamon

Instructions:

Core apples, sprinkle with cinnamon, and bake until tender.

Nutritional Information (per serving):

- Calories: 90
- Protein: 0.5g
- Potassium: 150mg
- Phosphorus: 10mg

Chia Seed Pudding with Berries:

Ingredients:

- Chia seeds
- Almond milk
- Mixed berries

Instructions:

Mix chia seeds with almond milk, refrigerate, and top with berries.

Nutritional Information (per serving):

- Calories: 120
- Protein: 3g
- Potassium: 100mg
- Phosphorus: 80mg

Frozen Banana Bites:

Ingredients:

- Banana slices
- Dark chocolate (melted)

Instructions:

Dip banana slices in melted dark chocolate and freeze.

Nutritional Information (per serving):

- Calories: 70
- Protein: 1g
- Potassium: 200mg

- Phosphorus: 20mg

Coconut Rice Pudding:

Ingredients:

- Arborio rice
- Coconut milk
- Vanilla extract

Instructions:

Cook rice in coconut milk, and sweeten it with vanilla extract.

Nutritional Information (per serving):

- Calories: 160
- Protein: 2g
- Potassium: 80mg
- Phosphorus: 40mg

Mango Sorbet:

Ingredients:

- Frozen mango chunks
- Water

Instructions:

Blend frozen mango with water until smooth.

Nutritional Information (per serving):

- Calories: 80
- Protein: 1g
- Potassium: 150mg
- Phosphorus: 10mg

Berries and Cream Parfait:

Ingredients:

- Mixed berries
- Whipped cream (unsweetened)

Instructions:

Layer berries with unsweetened whipped cream.

Nutritional Information (per serving):

- Calories: 90
- Protein: 1g
- Potassium: 100mg

- Phosphorus: 20mg

Peach and Almond Smoothie:

Ingredients:

- Fresh or frozen peaches
- Almond milk
- Vanilla protein powder (low-phosphorus)

Instructions:

Blend peaches with almond milk and protein powder.

Nutritional Information (per serving):

- Calories: 150
- Protein: 5g
- Potassium: 180mg
- Phosphorus: 60mg

Dark Chocolate Dipped Strawberries:

Ingredients:

- Fresh strawberries
- Dark chocolate (melted)

Instructions:

Dip strawberries in melted dark chocolate.

Nutritional Information (per serving):

- Calories: 60
- Protein: 1g
- Potassium: 100mg
- Phosphorus: 20mg

Chapter 7

Beverages for Kidney Health

Cucumber Mint Infused Water:

Ingredients:

- Cucumber slices

- Fresh mint leaves

Instructions:

Combine cucumber slices and mint leaves in water. Refrigerate for a refreshing drink.

Nutritional Information (per serving):

- Calories: 0

- Potassium: 10mg

- Phosphorus: 0mg

Herbal Iced Tea with Lemon:

Ingredients:

- Herbal tea bags

- Lemon slices

- Ice cubes

Instructions:

Brew herbal tea, chill, and serve over ice with lemon slices.

Nutritional Information (per serving):

- Calories: 0

- Potassium: 10mg

- Phosphorus: 0mg

Coconut Water and Pineapple Cooler:

Ingredients:

- Coconut water

- Pineapple chunks

- Ice cubes

Instructions:

Mix coconut water with pineapple chunks and serve over ice.

Nutritional Information (per serving):

- Calories: 60

- Potassium: 450mg

- Phosphorus: 30mg

Cranberry Lime Sparkler:

Ingredients:

- Unsweetened cranberry juice

- Lime juice

- Sparkling water

Instructions:

Mix cranberry and lime juice with sparkling water.

Nutritional Information (per serving):

- Calories: 20

- Potassium: 10mg

- Phosphorus: 5mg

Watermelon Basil Refresher:

Ingredients:

- Fresh watermelon cubes

- Fresh basil leaves

- Water

Instructions:

Blend watermelon cubes with fresh basil and strain. Serve chilled.

Nutritional Information (per serving):

- Calories: 30

- Potassium: 200mg

- Phosphorus: 10mg

Protein-Packed Shakes:

Almond Milk and Berry Smoothie:

Ingredients:

- Almond milk (unsweetened)

- Mixed berries

- Vanilla protein powder (low-phosphorus)

Instructions:

Blend almond milk, mixed berries, and protein powder until smooth.

Nutritional Information (per serving):

- Calories: 150

- Protein: 10g

- Potassium: 200mg

- Phosphorus: 80mg

Banana and Peanut Butter Protein Shake:

Ingredients:

- Banana

- Peanut butter (unsalted)

- Greek yogurt

Instructions:

Blend banana, peanut butter, and Greek yogurt for a creamy shake.

Nutritional Information (per serving):

- Calories: 200

- Protein: 15g

- Potassium: 300mg

- Phosphorus: 150mg

Avocado and Spinach Green Smoothie:

Ingredients:

- Avocado

- Baby spinach

- Almond milk

Instructions:

Blend avocado, baby spinach, and almond milk for a nutrient-rich smoothie.

Nutritional Information (per serving):

- Calories: 180

- Protein: 5g

- Potassium: 400mg

- Phosphorus: 80mg

Warm Beverages:

Ginger Turmeric Tea:

Ingredients:

- Fresh ginger

- Ground turmeric

- Hot water

Instructions:

Steep fresh ginger and turmeric in hot water for a soothing tea.

Nutritional Information (per serving):

- Calories: 0

- Potassium: 10mg

- Phosphorus: 0mg

Hot Lemon Honey Chamomile Tea:

Ingredients:

- Chamomile tea bags

- Lemon juice

- Honey (optional)

Instructions:

Brew chamomile tea, add lemon juice and honey to taste.

Nutritional Information (per serving):

- Calories: 10

- Potassium: 5mg

- Phosphorus: 0mg

Mocktails:

Virgin Mojito:

Ingredients:

- Fresh mint leaves

- Lime wedges

- Sugar substitute

- Soda water

Instructions:

Muddle mint leaves and lime wedges with a sugar substitute. Top with soda water.

Nutritional Information (per serving):

- Calories: 5

- Potassium: 20mg

- Phosphorus: 0mg

Berry Basil Lemonade:

Ingredients:

- Mixed berries

- Fresh basil leaves

- Lemon juice

- Sparkling water

Instructions:

Blend berries, basil, and lemon juice. Strain and mix with sparkling water.

Nutritional Information (per serving):

- Calories: 30

- Potassium: 40mg

- Phosphorus: 5mg

Dairy-Free Options:

Pineapple Coconut Smoothie:

Ingredients:

- Pineapple chunks

- Coconut milk (unsweetened)

- Ice cubes

Instructions:

Blend pineapple, coconut milk, and ice for a tropical smoothie.

Nutritional Information (per serving):

- Calories: 90

- Potassium: 170mg

- Phosphorus: 20mg

Raspberry Almond Milkshake:

Ingredients:

- Raspberries

- Almond milk (unsweetened)

- Almond extract

Instructions:

Blend raspberries, almond milk, and almond extract for a flavorful shake.

Nutritional Information (per serving):

- Calories: 80

- Potassium: 120mg

- Phosphorus: 10mg

Decaffeinated Options:

Decaf Iced Coffee with Vanilla Almond Milk:

Ingredients:

- Decaffeinated coffee

- Vanilla almond milk (unsweetened)

- Ice cubes

Instructions:

Brew decaf coffee, cool, and mix with vanilla almond milk over ice.

Nutritional Information (per serving):

- Calories: 20

- Potassium: 50mg

- Phosphorus: 20mg

Chapter 8

Conclusion

In conclusion, this Stage 4 Kidney Disease Cookbook for Seniors strives to be a comprehensive and supportive resource for individuals navigating the dietary challenges associated with advanced kidney disease. Recognizing the importance of nutrition in managing kidney health, we have curated a collection of recipes that not only cater to the specific dietary needs of seniors but also aim to make the journey towards better renal function enjoyable and flavorsome.

Throughout this cookbook, we have addressed the dietary challenges seniors with Stage 4 Kidney Disease face, providing insights into low-potassium foods, low-phosphorus alternatives, smart sodium swaps, and the delicate balance of proteins, carbs, and fats. Emphasizing the significance of monitoring fluid intake, we've crafted a 28-day sample meal plan, offering a diverse range of breakfast, lunch, and dinner options, accompanied by wholesome snacks and beverages, to help individuals sustain a kidney-friendly lifestyle. Dining out strategies and practical tips have been woven into the fabric of this cookbook, recognizing that maintaining social connections and enjoying meals outside the home are integral components of a fulfilling life. Additionally, we've delved into the importance of nutrition in managing kidney health, underlining the role of mindful eating in supporting overall well-being.

The recipes provided are not just a compilation of ingredients and instructions; they are a testament to the possibility of savoring delicious meals while prioritizing kidney health. From nutrient-packed smoothies to flavorful entrees, each recipe is designed to cater to the specific nutritional requirements of seniors with Stage 4 Kidney Disease, ensuring a balance between taste and health.

As we conclude this cookbook, we hope that it serves as a valuable companion, offering not only delectable recipes but also fostering a positive and empowering attitude towards managing Stage 4 Kidney Disease. May these culinary creations contribute to the well-being, vitality, and joy of our seniors, encouraging them to savor the flavors of life while nurturing their kidney health.

Printed in Great Britain
by Amazon

41767050R00066